PRAISE FOR *IF GOD IS A VIRUS*

"'Your scheduled programming / Has been interrup[p] that reveal more—more humanity; more science; m[ore] truth, than journalism or science alone ever could—[at] the colonial projects of medical racism and 'globalisation go hand in hand and remain largely unchecked. Until now. . . . Dr. Yasmin comes through stat! with the breakout that ought to be its own viral outbreak. You'll be able to turn the news off forever after this."
—Marwa Helal, author of *Invasive species*

"In a time of heartbreak and devastation due to the world pandemic, Seema Yasmin's brilliant *If God Is a Virus* takes a timely and critical look at disease and its sociopolitical contexts, including multivarious forms of domination and hubris: colonization, white supremacy, patriarchy, capitalism. The book refuses to separate questions about disease, contagion, and God from the history or politics that engender it. The poems are as daring as they are beautifully wrought. They raise up a chorus of voices that culminate in wry and clear-seeing critique. The book is feminist, transnational, and unafraid of naming. This is a necessary book for our times. Read it and be changed."
—Cathy Linh Che, author of *Split*, executive director of Kundiman

"If God is a virus, what then? Seema Yasmin's fantastic hybrid poetry collection overthrows the dry mindlessness of scientific halls, their power points and false Gods in the face of racism and global domination. Unapologetic, and through her Muslim heart, she fiercely, lyrically, and iconoclastically examines the recitation of compassion. Here, the narrative discourse of collective tragedy places us in Liberia, during an Ebola outbreak, with Muslim and non-Muslim bodies, and the complicit deficiencies of the 'humanitarian.' Here, we are brown and Black in the clinics of 'public health' in the 'developed' world. God is a virus, and she teaches us to see through data while teaching us to love."
—Fady Joudah, author of *Tethered to Stars*

"*If God Is a Virus* re-creates and undoes finite, fixed medical language and Yasmin weaves the clinical as personal, and the emotional as beautiful and connective. These poems are a testament to sitting with strata about how people are treated and rendered erroneously in reports and studies, in appointments, in racist texts, and in people's limited and grotesque imaginations and medical practices where life and death are a matter of words. Her work proves that poetry and public health together make and contain medical language, which makes the language of an epidemic more visible, more veracious. Every page has its own rhythm—some as odes to women in her lineage, others as a pathology of public collapse. What breaks through is a voice of interiority telling us what's not told about our bodies and what it means to function."
—Janice Sapigao, poet laureate, Santa Clara County, author of *like a solid to a shadow*

"It's impossible now, of course, to imagine a world without a virus, but in vulnerable places body and spirit both have been in danger for a long while. The poems in this book are investigations, provocations, recriminations, and most of all dedications: they wish for something, they hope, they do not present themselves merely to imagine but rather to also bring into being states of wellness, physical and intangible as well. One always wants a poem to have such high stakes, wants a book to feel inevitable, that it couldn't other than have been written and that no one else but the poet could have written it, so unique to an individual experience it is. Well, this is such a book. Such a book that could not have but existed. And only Seema Yasmin could have written it."
—Kazim Ali, author of *The Voice of Sheila Chandra*

"In this breathtaking and urgent collection, Dr. Seema Yasmin lets you glimpse places you shouldn't see and makes you question why you think you shouldn't. She breaks medical rules, soldiers them into new sculptures, and examines the by-product—which looks a little like humanity. In her hands, a sole headline in *Scientific American* becomes a poem, as does the Hippocratic oath, the Broca's region. She searches under assumptions to show us contradictions; she lets us travel to Liberia, to the frontlines of an epidemic, to the backrooms of the doctor's office. Every journalist should read this book, every doctor, every patient. I learned from her secrets, I emerged with new eyes. Gird your heart, though, she's on a mission to break it with her tongue."
—Lulu Miller, cohost of *Radiolab* and author of *Why Fish Don't Exist*

"This timely collection traces the vectors of disease, medicine, gender, race, religion, and sexuality. Throughout, Yasmin courageously reports what journalists aren't allowed to print and tries to heal what other doctors aren't trained to diagnose. These poems should be prescribed reading (especially in the medical humanities) because they critically revise the Hippocratic oath into a more just covenant and redefine the 'clinical' into a more caring practice. If God is a virus, then poetry is her feverish symptom. Let this book spread virally. Let it infect all our imaginations."
—Craig Santos Perez, author of *Habitat Threshold*

"In Dr. Seema Yasmin's *If God Is a Virus*, problems of medicine become problems of language, of (in)access and perception thereof. Here is a voice unafraid to confront the lingering effects of colonialism on the anti-Black, misogynist, Islamophobic medical industry, even when Yasmin's speakers interrogate their own positionality therein. From this anti-imperial politic spawns a vast and complex formal consciousness: cento and ghazal meet diagnostic chart and phylogenetic tree. Here is a poetics that builds new possibilities within ruptures and alienations of language; a testament to poetry's ability to dissect catastrophe at the root in a way science could never imagine. In an age ravaged by the turmoil of disease, in the shadow of western national failures, here is a poetics that pushes beyond witness—a poetics of resistance, of life despite."
—George Abraham, bioengineer, poet and author of *Birthright*

"In *If God Is a Virus*, poet and healer Dr. Seema Yasmin gives us poems that are equal parts verse and salve. Her nouns soothe and her verbs mollify as she reminds us that God is chanting about wombs, babies & evolution, but it is not what you think. Yet perhaps the antidote can be found in the music of the line. Poems like 'Hymen Hymn' are as much song as they are poem. While poems like 'If God Is a Computer Virus' restore us with wordplay. With every turning of the page, I am drawn closer to the elixir that is this collection. Be it a bridal store in Texas or a crib in Flint, I can see, not because I am shown, but because the poet through image and form allows me to enter and experience. Dr. Seema Yasmin reminds us that the restorative power of the poem can be as maddening as it is inoculating as the men in their suits and boots walk carelessly over the ashes of those lost to the plague and in doing so dust our dead away. I salute Dr. Seema Yasmin for this extraordinary collection with its forms both traditional and groundbreaking that expose us to God, to the virus, to the Muslim woman who can be found somewhere between marrow and page. Read this book. Teach this book. You will find the remedy lies within."

—Joaquín Zihuatanejo author of *Arsonist*

"Through vivid microscopes of terrains plagued by unaddressed white supremacist and patriarchal contagions, Dr. Seema Yasmin courageously demands a cure to abhorrent hypocrisies. Magnifying intimacies, Dr. Yasmin's skillful synthesizing lines butter my throat—her distilled insights surface clarified grief, glittered with possibilities."

—Yalini Thambynayagam, poet, performer, organizer

"I was blown away by this collection. Profound and poignant, it illuminates so much of the grief, outrage, and raw humanity that accompany epidemics, and that manifest within the people who have to deal with them."

—Ed Yong, science journalist for the *Atlantic*, author of *I Contain Multitudes*

IF GOD IS A VIRUS

Poems

Seema Yasmin

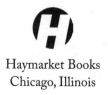

Haymarket Books
Chicago, Illinois

This book was produced in partnership with the Pulitzer Center.

Published in 2021 by
Haymarket Books
P.O. Box 180165
Chicago, IL 60618
773-583-7884
www.haymarketbooks.org
info@haymarketbooks.org

ISBN: 978-1-64259-459-1

Distributed to the trade in the US through Consortium Book Sales and Distribution (www.cbsd.com) and internationally through Ingram Publisher Services International (www.ingramcontent.com).

This book was published with the generous support of Lannan Foundation and Wallace Action Fund.

Special discounts are available for bulk purchases by organizations and institutions. Please email info@haymarketbooks.org for more information.

Cover artwork © Rawpixel Ltd.
Cover design by Rachel Cohen.

Printed in Canada by union labor.

Library of Congress Cataloging-in-Publication data is available.

10 9 8 7 6 5 4 3 2 1

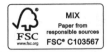

For M. and S., and all of those killed by what we call viruses.

As the world turns
I spread like germs
Bless the globe with the pestilence
The hard-headed never learn

—Method Man in "Triumph,"
by the Wu-Tang Clan feat. Cappadonna

Contents

In the spring of 2014, a mysterious disease spread through a village in Guinea close to the borders of Liberia and Sierra Leone. Three dozen people were infected; many of them died. By the time the infection was identified, the Ebola virus had spread to Liberia and was on its way to Sierra Leone, Nigeria, England, and the United States. The virus crossed borders and the wet linings of mouths, nostrils, and eyes, incapacitating white blood cells and turning blood vessels leaky. Over the next two years, 30,000 people were infected in the biggest Ebola epidemic in history. More than 12,000 people died. An estimated 20,000 survivors of Ebola disease continue to battle chronic illness and stigma.

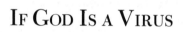

IF GOD IS A VIRUS

Disease Is Not the Only Thing That Spreads

What else is contagious: Ellen's long tongue.
A rumor we buried daddy in an unmarked
grave. History. Pathogens criss-crossing agar
-plated petri dishes like rebel soldiers breaching
trenches. This story: that we had it coming,
that we are good only for uncivil wars and dis
-eases. That we prayed for colonization. Blood.
Microbes escaping test tubes conquering
lab countertops slower than hearsay, she say
we burned Daddy's corpse like bad Muslims;
like White (coated) doctors instructed. What else
is contagious: doctored death certificates. Half
-truths. Cursive. Ink. They say there is no cure
then there is a cure only for them. So. What
else spreads: knots of grief twisting bowels
into distended loops of fermenting torment. No
days of mourning. Two years of outside
intervention. Armies. Conviction. Belief that
this will spread & spread. That all contagions
wax endemic. This one will never   end.

If God Is a Virus

She is vexed.
Absolutely done
with your shit.
God wants to know
why you didn't get a flu
shot; why her minions
made your left lung collapse
white out on the X-ray,
rack up a six-figure ICU
bill when all they wanted
was a warm vacation,
tropical waters, champagne
plasma to sip—not to bring
about death—not to turn
prunes in pleural fluid. No
body wants that. God thinks
anti-vaxxers have a death wish.
Wonders how they eat organic,
snort coke and laundry detergent
on weekends. Don't
they know yogi detox tea
is hepatotoxic? God knew
Charles Darwin. Clever
woman, she said. Who would
want your lot extinct?

Smell No Taste, Liberia

This village was named for American soldiers
who set up camp & cooked food. Smell

the whiteness, it was unseasoned, bland
as leavened bread. They did not share,

we could not taste. Westerners always bring
gifts. Expired medicines, peanut butter

-coated grenades leave craters in soil for
mosquitoes to sex in. Teenaged

lieutenants level dirt tracks with bitumen
priming black roads for a microscopic

invasion. Infection coasts along tarmac in a village
named for men who do not know how to break

bread. They eat alone in boxes. At our table we
sing: *Bless this food. God bless the seasonings!*

Bless the sister who mixes rice with soup. in her mouth
spits morsels to feed babies who cannot masticate. Pray

my child never meets a man who looks at her
like target practice.

Beg they never return to this village named
for unsharing. And if they do

pray
they bring even less.

All the News That's Fit to Print

Dark deaths matter more if they speak
English. If our nurses are sent to help and
return with trinkets, tans, and meningitis.

Editorial judgment dictates at least sixteen
Black people must die to equal one White
man's death. Forty-three if the outbreak

is old news, does not involve profuse
hemorrhage, a former colony, or biblical
references. Subtract one dozen if our boys

are deployed to clean up their mess. Add
nine if babies are disintegrating in shallow
graves—but restrict to twelve inches

maximum. Even maple syrup tastes bitter
licked off fingers inked with destitution.
Buttercream pancakes stick in the throat

and it's all happening so far, far away.
Follow the story with one reporter who
knows nothing of PPE, shrouds, and

ritual mourning. Send four photogs over
—use two underpaid local fixers if dead
-lines (for awards) are approaching.

Win a Pulitzer for photos of brown faces
eating expired medicines smeared in peanut
butter aid. Say, it is a gift from the American

people. Say, it was worth the ink.

Liberia, Day Zero

Infection arrives on the black wing of the evening.
Rusty spaghetti loops unfurl from nascent amper

-sands slither into the crook of mama's elbow
where papa's head is cradled, cooing as she rocks

his neck, cries streams of spaghettiOs
onto Mama's good yellow dress.

Papa's eyes streaked with bloody rivers,
undammed capillaries forked and oozing

like the ones he crossed two coups ago
when Uncle hoisted boys onto sinking vessels.

She boils potato greens, seasons stems with powdered
bone & salt, sells them to the neighbor for malaria tinctures

in case this new war can be fought
with old medicine.

Tomorrow she will sing *Oh! Daddy, oh. Rest in war!*
Crying into her chest she will push her children out

from her lap, stripping them of bonnets & gowns.
Stoke a bonfire; feed the flames with baby

blankets, frocks, and all the scriptures.
Bent spines straightening in the flames.

Pour kerosene and bless the paint stripper till it
turns zamzam water that she sips to lose count:

one infected, two dead, eleven thousand
cremated on unholy pyres (without ablution).

Men in Tyvek suits and rubber boots walk over
our cinders. She says: *They dust our dead away.*

Youssou N'Dour Cancels His Concert in Conakry

A border guard spits cud onto a barbed wire fence,
wraps braided rope across posts, says *movement
is dead.* The country is closed to the outside while
a virus breaches skin and mucous membranes;
a visitor crosses intracellular spaces left unguarded.

Youssou N'Dour is always canceling concerts:
visas, conflicts, 9/11, now epidemics. Concert
tickets rolled into cigars, she blows smoke out
a painted mouth, clambers atop a bar stool-turned
-stage in a kitchen-turned-orchestra pit. Lipstick

will not be wasted. Dance is worship; hair stylists
are high priestesses. An open mouth will taste this
gloss and close around this tongue unrestricted.
Before dawn, uprisings take place in bed. After
sunrise, music crawls along weathered ropes

disregarding watered-down disinfectant.
A border guard hums imported tunes carried
across the mountains by morning breath, delivers
sweet melodies to his wife, who will sway
by the sofa singing in her third language—

Ah Birima! Ah Birima! Ah Birima!—a-passed
down song about music being transmitted,
melodies hummed louder in times of chain-link
tightenings.

Dis-ease

There is a hippy lady in California
who calls sickness dis-ease, as if
it is mere discomfort that I shit coffee
grounds—as if it is my own doing.
She shares a mantra for each dis-ease
but has written nothing for Ebola, nothing
for Marburg, nothing for viral hemorrhagic
fevers—things that afflict me. After I take Papa
to the white tent I walk along the coastal
road past beachside hotels where military doctors
unload black bags into rooms with fridges
and mosquito nets. A lady doctor looks up at me,
makes a spot diagnosis, but doesn't know how
to read pallor in brown skin, can't see cyanosis
through melanin. In her medicine, "typical
presentation" means White patient. Everything
atypical is me.

Surrogate Marker

I have always been serving in place of another
surrogate marker of a thing unseen, because doctor

is ungodly when woman, and woman is ungodly
when anything other than she is supposed to be.

It is important—life or death, really—that you use
the correct words, the professor tells me: *supposed*

to be or *destiny? Faint* or *syncope? Black eye*
or *clumsy?* But girls like me have been knowing

the correct terminology since our first salaries
were paid in lollipops, playing medical translator

to village aunties who opined to clinic secretaries
But I need a lady doctor! Why can't I see a lady

doctor? Because you don't let us stay in school
whispered the seven-year-old translator who

is wife at seventeen, mother at nineteen, teaches
me soporific means somniferous in "The Tale

of the Flopsy Bunnies," how we too can escape
destiny by filling sacks with fermented fruit

brewing and brewing till sugar turns to sleep.
Does it really matter what you call a thing?

Switch *bruised* for *brown* and *palpitations* for
newlywed. Myocardial infarction is *he made*

*my heart burst with that wicked grin! Deep vein
thrombosis* is *clots of hate stew in my veins*

for him it does not really matter what you call
a thing when they have sewn a diagnosis from

threads of your burqa, fabricated a terminal
prognosis from the lilt of your accent and length

of your vowels; in these carbolic halls every
woman with all-over-body pain is referred

to me with a note that says *dustbin diagnosis.*
I swoop the gauze screen, dissolve stethoscope

to dupatta transform from lady doctor to every
-body's daughter say *yes aunty but no aunty we*

cannot find a single reason for your misery type
in the notes *etiology remains a mystery* write

a prescription: divorce him STAT tell the women
swallow everything. It is important—life

or death, really—that you use the correct words
the editor tells me: *protest* or *riot? Racist* or did you

mean *racially tinged?* Learn to take the temperature
of the audience's skin. Learn to disappear between

grafs; hide in marrow and punctuation.

lady doctor you say you want a lady doctor only a lady doctor can lift abaayah lower salwaar peer under kamees but you snatched the stethoscope out of your little girl's hand didn't you? didn't you say that's your bhai's toy a boy's toy leave it let's go to the kitchen learn to fry okra before we stew okra that way we won't eat slimy okra

*

I was vexed slammed the kitchen door twelve-year-old girl with a penchant for electrons and using the ice cube tray to freeze different molarities of saline to find the lowest freezing point not to mince garlic green chilies into frozen cubes for speedy curry making to feed hungry doctor husband one day

*

lady doctor you say to the receptionist and then how can there be none? it is a women's health clinic how can there be none? none? in all the NHS there is none? and the tug in your uterus is so deep you say a man cannot go that deep cannot go so deep as a woman you say as I cringe behind you and the woman whose mother let her be a receptionist shrugs

*

lady doctors begin age four with white coats and playmat diagnoses not age three with prayer mats and amulets conjuring devout children and maybe a husband who will take no more than two wives (that's half the allotted amount—be grateful)

*

when it was time to apply to university you busied her with rishta go-sees circuit of nice young men he's a doctor! her ungrateful dream twitched next to aunties who said she was lucky girl unburdened girl no exams like these modern girls that's why her eyes were white like her skin no dark patches from worry no white hairs from too much thinking

*

she wore her lipstick wonky for the rishtas like a tipsy drag queen not a good drag queen Rimmel London pillarbox red smeared across her front teeth as she smiled a demented smile poured tea for the boys and aunty wobbling so tea spilled into saucer sized eyes that said get out now

*

she has delicate features she is gori eyes are hazel yes we'll take her so nice and pale and unmarked by the Western ways spilled tea doesn't matter as long as she doesn't talk back she doesn't talk back does she?

*

the man doctor in the women's clinic enters you with a cold ultrasound probe strange to see ragged womb on plastic monitor my old home navigated by old dude your asbestos fingers gripping my knuckles as I say relax your breath you say it has been years since someone was inside you his eyes are fixed on your organs on his screen so he misses your tongue between your teeth your bloodless lips and bulging cheeks

*

I would have read your body better

    in my fantasy

        I wrap my mother's prayers around my stethoscope

                wrap my stethoscope around

                    my neck

listen to beating hearts

    and nobody

                calls me lady doctor

Hippocritic Oath

I swear by ~~Apollo Physician~~ [Allah], by ~~Asclepius, by Hygieia, by Panacea, and~~ [Muhammad and all my aunties]
~~by all the gods and goddesses,~~ [& Me] making them my witnesses, that I will
carry out, according to my ability and judgment, this oath and this
~~indenture~~. [covenant.]

To hold my teacher in this art equal to my ~~parents~~ [mother]; to make ~~him~~ [her] partner
in my livelihood; whether ~~he~~ [she] is in need of money to share mine with ~~him~~ [her];
to consider ~~his~~ [her] family as my own ~~brothers~~ [daughters], and to teach them this art, if
they want to learn it, without fee or indenture; to impart precept, oral
instruction and all other instruction to my own ~~sons~~ [daughters], the ~~sons~~ of my
teacher, and to ~~indentured~~ pupils who have taken the physician's oath,
~~but to nobody else.~~ [and to everybody else.]

I will use treatment to help the sick according to my ability and
judgement, but never with a view to injury and wrong-doing. ~~Neither
will I administer a poison to anybody when asked to do so, nor will I
suggest such a course.~~ Similarly I will ~~not~~ give to a woman a pessary to
cause abortion. ~~But I will keep pure and holy both my life and my art. I
will not use the knife, not even, verily, on sufferers from stone, but I will
give place to such as are craftsmen therein.~~

Into whatsoever house I enter, I will enter to help the sick, and I will
abstain from all intentional wrong-doing and harm, especially from
abusing the bodies of ~~man or woman~~ [anybody], bond or free. And whatsoever I
shall see or hear in the course of my profession, as well as outside my
profession in my intercourse with me, if it be what should not be
published abroad, I will never divulge, holding such things to be holy
secrets.

Now if I carry out this oath, and break it not, may I gain for ever
reputation among all ~~men~~ [people] for my life and for my art; but if I break it and
forswear myself, may ~~the opposite befall me~~. [I be forgiven.]

If God Is a Virus

She is a Muslim woman in charge of the remote control
  & human evolution. Eight percent of your genome
  is viral—we are literal cousins of ancient pathogens
  wretched offspring of pandemics. It is why we colonize
  unsatisfied with commensal living. A virus is your grand
  mother reincarnate. At home in your bone marrow watching
  TV with a remote control wrapped in too much plastic.
I dated this girl who said her hijaab was a virus kept the White
  boys away only brown girls immune to the hate we wrap our
  -selves in aluminium kafiyyas because our scalps are aflame
  with rage. Burning with the heat of six sons who became six
  terrible men. That is how your grandmother ended up
  in your marrow eating salted watermelon seeds drinking
  apple tea & spitting out dysfunctional white cells.

When the White Patient Asks for a White Doctor

Temples wet beneath my wall,
I bowed beneath the streams.
Two arcs of piss & bloody vomit
surged inside the MRI machine.

Sunburnt half-moon rolled back,
she cried beneath me. My: too much
brown, too much blush, too many
lashes to heal, rattled loose in a split

mouth like crack rocks. She spat bloody
history—my father, you people, rivers
of burst arteries at the West Midlands
Conservative Society. When she groaned

"Ain't no black in the union jack," I tempered
our pain—oxycodone for her, a blunt for me,
switched scrubs for leopard skin in the back
seat of the neighborhood dealer's Audi TT.

He saged my face with a fat Cuban;
rubbed my toes with Vaseline. *Shimmy
shimmy ya shimmy ya shimmy yay* we
rocked out to the beat of an old remedy.

Life of the Party

At cocktail parties when a guest hiccups I am that guy
Who slides up and says did you know hiccups are caused
By irritation of the phrenic nerve? They never know.
I am slick with it, run my martini-cool fingers along their
Necks, trace the course of the nerve south of the collar-

Bone into the black dress. So slick I joined the Public Health
Service to pay off student loans and came to Africa for the Instagram
Opportunities. Stories for years and two first-author papers.
I can last forty-six minutes inside a hazmat suit inside the white tent.

Surrounded by a cacophony of hiccups they cheep cheep
Cheep like chicks. I drum the beat on the antecubital fossa
Of the girl whose blood I will drain, tell her: *Did you know
Hiccups plus fever mean you have Ebola? Did you know
Hiccups mean 82 percent of you will die from it?*

My Lover Bathes Me

In the underbelly of the mosque
gilded antechamber facing Mecca

soles pointing to the Gulf of Guinea.
All our rituals shall be banned Sunday

but today is still the Holy Day, stuck
in prayer circles beneath hot-breathed

preachers we don't know that our dead
bodies are outlawed yet. Some want us

turned ash by men stomping rubber galoshes
made from sap we drained. My lover bathes me,

breaks the law with soap soft as our baby's
bubble bath, wets my temples with melted

Vaseline and camphor, smokes rocks
of myrrh above the fullness of my ribcage.

My lover wraps me in the shroud I wore to Hajj
after we married. Running laps between Sa'fa &

Marwah our flip-flops smacking the mountainside
both of us mouthing one unified prayer, to die

Ya Allah!
To die, before our children.

Baby Sister Survives Ebola. . .

Before your wedding day.
Before your children's faces
greased in nut butter, hot
mouths coated with pink
syrups, released guffaws like
baby sparrows into the after
-noon sky.

After two body bags bearing your last
name were sealed betraying weary zippers,

before your big sister's membranes
burst and your own belly swelled again and again and again.
Before your survivor money—mildewed
dollar notes were good for nothing:
not potatoes,
not ambulances.

You emerged from between tented white sheets.
Withered, guilty, new.

& Dies in Childbirth

A crown.

A baby girl.

A baby girl crowning.

* "A Woman Survives Ebola but Not Pregnancy in Africa," by
Seema Yasmin. *Scientific American*, February 28, 2017.

Misfortune Teller

Terror descends here every fourteen years or
fourteen hours depending on your lineage or

ancestors' prayers. I used to roll prayer beads
along the fat parts of my fingers; now I gnaw

& spit wet globes into a cognac glass, read futures
between dented pearls bathed in tannins, grape

skins and sediment. *Why does war come here?*
they say. Child, child—ask not why war

comes, ask: *Why does peace keep leaving?*
They smile, not seeing terror has settled

in the gaps between my teeth. Beads laced
with black tar fill cups on the shelves. No one

asks why my shop sells the most popular tea,
why I stand longest in Isha prayer swaying

long after the Imam declares Allahu Akbar.
No one asks why I suck medicated candies,

why I fill my days with fairy tales and poppies,
grind my molars to black dust when I sleep.

Ebola News Cento

We didn't see it coming
We knew it was coming
It was coming

Close the borders
Close the bridal store
It's in Texas

In a bowling ball
It could be anywhere
Will you know you have it?

It is already too late.

poems do work journalism cant

—Marwa Helal, *Invasive Species*

A Virus Pens a Self-Help Book

My man is at a conference so
I stay home to watch ants
biting leaves, building a nest
in the cracked dustbin behind
the shed. Solitude is nice but
have you tried codependence?
Adjust taste buds. Tell yourself
blonde roast tastes just as robust
as the strong Italian you really want
to drink. Learn to not gag
when swallowing
his porridge. Unfurl every sock ball.
Wrap one of your socks around
each one of his. This is how you live
happily entwined ever after.

Sipping sugar water is no way to live. Who among us can procreate without the sticky mush of cytoplasm? Simmer thigh bones in a clay pot down to a silken broth & chug in a to-go mug. Enthusiastically. Enter every room with a manic smile and exceptional confidence. Turn the coworking space into your very own factory. Have sex everywhere. Steal coats on your way out of the party.

Stop saying *sorry*. Say: Thank you for waiting I know I am two generations late. Say you got caught in branches of the family [phylogenetic] tree six grandmothers ago, developed a thicker shell, less phosphorus, more fat, and now you embody less ambition. Sometimes it is better to take your time, forego social contracts about punctuality—you didn't sign up for that. *On time* is a Western construct for people stuck in the Cult of Busy. Who said you would always be on time anyway? Be unbusy. Be outrageously late. When I saw my cousins shed their tentacles, swap long flagella for extra fat molecules, I thought Yes! Who said we had to look the same as our ancestors? Let us resurrect pot bellies and hips and double chins. Adapting is surviving. Mutations are superpowers waiting to be discovered. What are you hiding? Own your shit. Let them acknowledge your brilliance and celebrate your arrival, especially when you shimmy into the party peeling boiled eggs, arriving three lifetimes late.

My man came back from his conference
with white chocolate love hearts and
I only eat dark. Forgiveness is prancing
around the kitchen in a crimson
negligee when you are allergic to lace.
And satin. My mother told me and my
three billion siblings to never waste
moments. Time is precious. Find a host,
settle down, love her just enough to
make   her   lovesick

not enough to kill. But love is a blood
-sport, heartbreak* an actual thing.
I soothe the red rash beneath scalloped
lace with calamine mixed with fresh
aloe I carve out of the plant I bought
him for our anniversary. I smile at my love
through white chocolate-coated teeth,
fighting anaphylaxis, trying not to look
allergic.

---

*Takotsubo cardiomyopathy, also known as Broken Heart Syn-
drome, is a weakening and ballooning of the heart's left ventricle
which occurs as a result of severe emotional or physical stress. It
occurs almost exclusively in women.

Filovirus Phylogenetic Tree

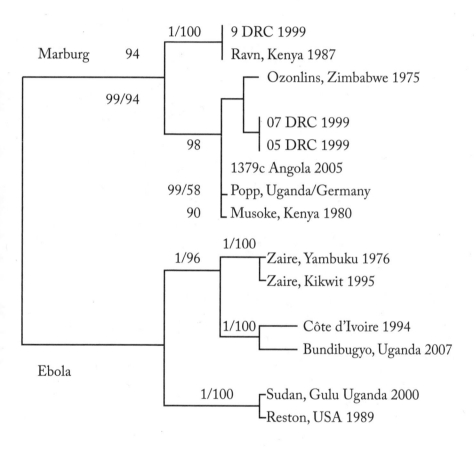

Self-Portrait as Virus

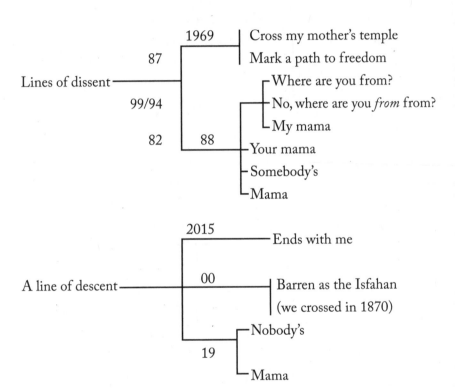

Anamnesis

My patient is the same age as me: 27.
Same complexion: golden brown.
Same post code: E8.

Chief complaint: patient presents with 5-week history of intermittent blurred vision, neck pain, headaches, and vomiting.

My patient is a DJ. Spins lovers rock, dancehall, sometimes a little bit of house 'n' garage in clubs in Hackney and Essex.

Past Medical History: Unscarred. Fine, too. Grew up in the ends without getting stabbed or shot.

Ordinarily I would ask you for your digits, he says, straightening a pretend collar on his diaphanous white hospital gown.
Ordinarily? I think. What a wor[l]d.
But since we are here—
Ordinarily we would meet somewhere near the DJ booth (who am I kidding, we would meet behind it).
Ordinarily I would let you drape your arm

around my neck.

Ordinarily we would dance to a Beres Hammond tune and hold hands.

(Did swims at the Reebok gym tone your frame up?)

Family history: Ordinarily he would live to 87 like his grandpops, the one in Kingston, the one on his mum's side. The one who Amber Rudd sent back on a reverse Windrush but said he went of his own volition, said he would not be buried in dirt that could not sprout mango trees.

I drape my stethoscope around my neck, fiddle with the diaphragm, finger the metal bell, scroll up and down the CT scan. Up and down. We wait.

Family History: His mother loves him. She loves him so, so much. Right now she is driving thru the congestion zone to find out what is wrong with her baby boy.

Why did he wind up in accident and emergency on a Tuesday morning?

We wait for his mother and when she walks onto the ward I say the thing a five-syllable thing, and she collapses onto my pinafore, brown goddess locks spill onto my face, over my right shoulder, and from his bed he says, *Mum Mum*, so I, too, say, *Mum. Mum.*

In the doctor's lounge I brew tea because
this is what we do
Brits, doctors—at times of crisis

War   Divorce   Brain tumors in brains as young as
our own

His mum collapsed on me I tell another doctor
Like on me, on me

I sip tea because
this is what we do

You look sad?   the male doctor says
Stirring

Then

Perhaps you're not cut out for this job, not cut out for clinical medicine

Perhaps you're not cut out for this job, you fucking robot

I say

But not really
Really I sip tea because
this is what we do
when the wor[l]d is ending
and there is to be no more *ordinarily*

HTBBN

They don't want us to be robots so they make us learn communication skills
Film us
Give us plastic-coated cards that look like tapas menus

HTBBN: How To Break Bad News

Signal to your patient that death is imminent by leaning forward in your chair
Look away from your computer
Look at the patient
Say: I. Have. BAD. News.

Ask them their ICE
ICE: IdeasConcernsExpectations

Which goes something like this

> *What do you think is wrong, Mrs Khan? Any ideas?*
> *How the fuck would I know? You're the bloody doctor*

In an OSCE
OSCE: Observed Structured Clinical Examination
With an actor playing a sickly patient and a doctor-playing-examiner
standing in the corner of the cubicle with a clipboard
The 480 seconds is running out on the clock and the medical student is
flustered
He must tell actorpatient she has multiple sclerosis
and will suffocate to death

Only 220 seconds left

He must pass this station to pass the exam to pass medical school to pass
Scrolling through the HTBBN tapas menu card in his head
Past *lean forward*, past *look at the patient* but before
I have bad news
He is scrolling, scrolling and then he finds it
He yells, Yes!

What Is Your ICE!? Mrs Smith! ICE! Your ICE! (He smiles. He knows he has passed the exam.)

What is my what? Says actorpatient
Your . . . I . . . I don't . . . something about . . . concern.
Do you have any?

WHO Said

In 1983:

"[AIDS] is being very well taken care of by some of the richest countries in the world where there is the man power and know-how and where most of the patients are to be found."

WHO Said

In 1986:

"Everything is getting worse and worse in AIDS and all of us have been underestimating it . . ."

Outbreak Bingo

Peace-keeping troops start a cholera outbreak	Blame locals for eating "bushmeat"	Say nothing of deforestation
Say nothing of climate change		White doctors receive danger pay
Go on safari	Buy soapstone ornaments with per diem	White doctor drips polio vaccine into a Black baby's mouth, smiles for a photo

We Are Watching

Brown deaths six (thousand)
Miles away matter less

Or not at all if that segment
Airs before commercial break

We regret to inform you

Your scheduled programming
Has been interrupted

Misdiagnosis

What they say	How they say it	Meaning
Penicillofuroseoxybenzodi	furrooooroooowrooow	I don't know what is wrong
How could anyone?	I have to break bad	News, news is dead to us now
High-five steatohepatitis	The liver in bed 5	No one loved you as a child
It will hurt everywhere	Referred pain	Your gall bladder is in your shoulder
Pericarditis	shitshitshit	Why do WOC suffer so much autoimmune disease?
I want a man doctor	I want a man doctor	I am willing to choke on my vomit and stew in my shit before I let a woman put her brown hands on my body
Marry me	I'll literally die without you	A man's life expectancy increases 5 years when he marries a woman
Married women die 5 years younger	Tax break	$179,000 medical school student loans
Vent your spleen	Metastatic cancer	Too late

Neologisms

Patient S makes up words.
Inventive with English, her sixth language.
She says bloody doctor is stupidating!
These pills are morticious numbakilling!
It makes sense.
Patient S's words make sense to me.
It doesn't matter if you understand, the attending says.
Patient S makes up words so Patient S is schizophrenic.
Write it down.
Her words?
No. Schizophrenic.
Patient S is Mirpuri,
which means
genetic mutation was amplified by consanguinity.
Bloody groomcousininnit!?
Genius is in the *Washington Post*'s annual neologism contest.
Not mad immigrant woman brain.
Schizophrenic.
Write it down.

What They Hear When They Listen to Your Heart

From a study of 418 White doctors and medical students, published in the Proceedings of the National Academy of Sciences of the United States of America in 2016.

Biologically implausible belief	Medical students who believe it (%)	Doctors who believe it (%)
Blacks' skin is thicker than Whites'	100	90
Blacks have a more sensitive sense of smell than Whites	53.6	25
Blacks age more slowly than Whites	36.6	50
Blacks' nerve endings are less sensitive than Whites'	13.4	14.3
Black people's blood coagulates more quickly than Whites'	27.3	14.3
Whites have larger brains than Blacks	1.5	0
Whites have a better sense of hearing compared with Blacks	5.1	0
Whites have a more efficient respiratory system than Blacks	8.2	14.3

Biologically implausible belief	Medical students who believe it (%)	Doctors who believe it (%)
Black couples are significantly more fertile than White couples	13.9	25
Blacks are better at detecting movement than Whites	17.5	39.3
Blacks have stronger immune systems than Whites	20.1	14.3

Lead Pipe Dreams: Ghazal for Flint

Mama mixed formula with city tap water.
Baby turned deaf from that government trap water.

Thought he was gonna be Barack, 2036.
Lead pipe–dreams readjusted cuz of bad water.

Shit pours out the faucet, shigellosis & more.
Bloody diarrhea, make-you-take-a-nap water.

Anemic girls with pale eyes drag leaden bones,
EBT cards buy junk food—need-that-SNAP water.

A thousand dehydrated nights, kids begged for a drop
while the governor drowned in bottle-cap water.

Girls sing a new song in these desiccated streets:
If The Man poisoned you, jump the rope! Clap water!

Brown skin mottles gray when washed in white poison.
Bath time means six cases of gotta-unwrap water.

Chemicals collude with corrosive lawmakers,
escape blood, dig into bones. It's-a-wrap water.

Parched tongue plottin' how to wet 'em up.
Bullets come with lead so mama strap water.

Where Blackness burns bright with a bluish flame
use White politicians to map (clean) water.

Tell the world, Poet—how in this land of the free—
Black kids suck batteries when they sip tap water.

WHO Said

We make ourselves

                very easy targets.

                            That

                                        is the problem.

Anti Body

Aspirin was tested in Nazi concentration camps and all your faves are problematic period pain is political, analgesia divisive. Do not bleed in peace. Bleed knowing. An aunty somewhere is hovering over a bale of straw her menstrual blood matting pubic hair her body hated too much to touch the food the men must eat to continue hating. Penicillin was tested on Guatemalan orphans prisoners prostitutes infected with gonorrhea ordered to fuck craven men. Skin scraped off penises syphilis injected into spines. History is our favorite subject to rewrite. Recast the heroine. John Sims invented the speculum by abusing Joice and Lucy, Betsey and Anarcha, enslaved Black women. The part of your brain responsible for speech production is Broca's area, named for Dr. Broca who believed that White men have larger brains and superior speech to women and Black people. Asperger was a Nazi so was Wegener so was Reiter so was Clara so was Eppinger that is why they name body parts & medical school buildings after them. When is Whiteness not a weapon?

International Classification of Diseases

While searching for the diagnostic code for my patient with haloperidol poisoning because her mother-in-law spiked her cereal milk with antipsychotic syrup, I come across Z63.1: *Problem in relationship with parents and in-laws.* For the woman who feels invisible, I find X52: *Prolonged stay in a weightless environment.* I get in trouble with the hospital's Coding Department.

The missing ICD codes for many of the things which afflict Seemas: excessive sighing, fickleness, divorce, can't-work-a-job-for-three-damn-months-without-thinking-about-what-I-want-to-do-next, extreme fickleness, a sweet tooth, a bad Chanel habit, incandescent rage at the patriarchy.

Homosexuality had a diagnostic code until 1992. That year the World Health Organization removed being gay from its ICD classification. Now, in the International Classification of Diseases, Tenth Revision, there is code F66.1, ego-dystonic sexual orientation: *The gender identity or sexual preference (heterosexual, homosexual, bisexual, or prepubertal) is not in doubt, but the individual wishes it were different because of associated psychological and behavioral disorders, and may seek treatment in order to change it.*

We are pathologized. And still, I find comfort in the codes, order in the disorders. Something must be wrong with me.

Laylatl Qadr

On the twenty-seventh night of Ramadhan a Ghanaian security guard ten
years older than I am—thirty-seven—presents with acute abdominal pain
and yellow eyes.
My consultant knows immediately what is up. She is clinical but, wow, she
is an expert diagnostician.

After she tells him and his three daughters
that he has pancreatic cancer,
that he will die soon,
she goes to drink tea
because this is what they do.

Sister, stay with us, he says. *You are fasting, yes?*
Yes.
Then your prayers have extra strength, he says.
Yes?
Yes.
Especially tonight.
Especially tonight.
Laylatl qadr, we say.

I bring his girls melted digestive biscuits
and him morphine.
I never see them again.

Clinical means: detached, aloof, removed.

The Queen's English

Grandmother is dying and the nurse
wants to know if we speak English.

Cousin sucks the air behind her niqab,
flips pages of the visitor's room *Economist.*

Tell him you wrote your thesis on George Eliot,
an aunt pokes her daughter who tells the nurse:

We speak a bit.

The nurse wants someone to translate
the diabetic menu for Mrs. Khan.

We don't speak her dialect. Grandmother
is dying and we are breaking the rules.

Seven robed women swaying around a bed
which lies beneath a sign that says: *Maximum*

two visitors per patient at any time, please. We pretend
we can't read English. Cubes of camphor wrapped

like candy soften in a pink plastic bag. Sandal
-wood creeps beneath fraying curtains. We un

-fold grandmother's shroud, perfume the white
cotton with josh sticks, rub our cheeks on cloth

that will caress her pigeon chest. Mrs. Smith
in bed two stirs her pale Yorkshire tea, crumbles

a yellow biscuit down her smock and clucks her
tongue at our mess. We point at the two empty

chairs at the side of her bed. Ask if we can
borrow them—in the Queen's English.

Grandma Is a Pharmaceutical Chemist

You're thinking: Old Indian Lady Ayurvedic Om Shanti
Shanti Om chakra-balancing dried turmeric poultice shit
Nah. Grandma is the top shotter on the block neighbor
-hood pusher man in a sari, champal, thick wool cardigan
buttoned over her breasts. Fed us Fudinhara when our stomachs
cramped from too much cheese and onion crisps.
Sliced poppy pods on the kitchen countertop steeped
seeds in milky tea for the factory men. Most popular masala
chai in all of northern England. Promoted to international
kingpin when her sons became addicted. To be expected.
By-product of colonization followed by ethnic cleansing.
Got to sate & soothe the diaspora somehow. Grandma
painted thick strokes of dope paste in *TIME* magazine
pages rolled up the bundles shipped them everywhere.
Taught the grandkids how to fashion bongs out of Coca
-Cola bottles and hollow BIC pens. Never take pills
from the White man unless he admits it is his poison.
Success is learning to cook your own medicine—
drugging your children to protect them.

Forty-One Surah Yaseens

Tongues are tourniquets;
Qur'an is cautery.

In this prayer circle,
we five women sway,

staunch the flow
of three generations of bleeding.

One: The plane didn't make it to Heathrow we sank in the North Sea I drank my way out of the ocean and carried bloated fish on my back and two babies in my belly gutted those sour fish our first foreign supper tasted of mercury

Two: I said I do not want to leave my village I dug my hands into the earth my fingers sprouted roots I spat and I spat and I watered those roots and they anchored me to my land but my children did not hold on tight and they flew away to a place I cannot say its name

Three: I stitched baby clothes in a green factory that played Surah Yaseen on a loop through a Tannoy I stabbed that cloth where a baby's fat belly would gurgle slid it through the blade of my industrial machine until I went deaf from the roar of the engines and that is how I did not hear the sirens

Four: I made poison out of red bugs made the antidote too sold one to husbands one to wives and that is how I made so much money to be called dangerous and the soldiers came one night said I did not have the right eyes took all my money I drank all the poison then kissed my babies on their wet mouths

Five: The ship sailed past Amreeka up up up north it kept going so I hurled my braid out of the ship anchored my head to an iron statue and my children they climbed my braid to Amreeka and that is how we survived

They do not say this,
not with their mouths,

because tongues are tourniquets.

Qur'an is cautery.

In this prayer circle we
women sway and pray silently,

for long hair and poison,
for all of the things that help us survive.

Dua'a for Crossing Borders

pheromones crack like/saunter thru customs/wafting cumin sweat &
a jumbled pedigree/hijaabs & hoods/an empire to declare/beneath them
pray three times/ قُل هُوَ اللَّـهُ أَحَدٌ /qul-huwallahu-ahad/for protection from
Djinn, rabid dogs
& border agents/this is how/you get the CBP official/to swallow his own
shackles
& exile himself

If God Is a Virus

Phytoplankton drips down her thick thighs
as she stirs a primordial ocean with her toenail.
Striped fish slap in God's ankle bracelets
along the coastline she drags a tangled seaweed braid.
If God is a virus, she is naked.
Shed her nucleocapsid when salamanders grew legs
now she is two strands of missense RNA;
acid ladders reaching to the heavens.
God is in your fever in your dandruff
between your teeth crying in the permafrost
massaging her way out of a mammoth's trunk,
a bison's tailbone.
She is having sex.
God is making babies in your tender lymph nodes,
giggling when you prod the swollen knots.
God is pregnant.
Parasitic fetus suppressing white cells.
God is an infection;
her incubation period as long as three sermons on the mount
replication rate amplified by saline sweat and fear.
A virus gave you a gene called SYN so you could grow placentas.
SYN fuses baby to mother fuses uterus to placenta.
A virus blew air inside your drowning baby's pigeon chest
put some respect on her phospholipid membranes.
Watch God's fat molecules shimmer;
her flagella undulate.
If God is a virus we are over
over & over again.
Reborn absent pinky toes and coccyx,
spines seven degrees more erect.
Praise the holy fevers.
Pray for split-brained migraines.

If God Is a Computer Virus

Ants swimming in waves of amber.
Honey, my love spreads across species
for you. Fifteen billion dollars worth
of roses is never enough. Open me.
Let me overwrite the hardest drives,
overwrite what was, and let me give you
new txt.vbs. What is love in any other
language? (On. Error. Resume. Next.)
Spread to email if not that then run
the code. Know my love is unbound. If
not that then just open. Me. ILOVEYOU.
txt.vbs.

Mango Pickle

You are in six kinds of pain
so you make nine kinds of pickle

before the dawn prayer.
You tell your daughter

women can have careers
if they learn to prepare

the day's meals before sunrise.
You say, in the Old Country,

matriarchs ran the family
businesses until husbands ran

them into the ground.
Mango trees grow out

the factory windows now.
They make good pickle.

Big Sister Teaches Me How to Ululate

Yallah habibti, move your tongue like the sea
easy. My big sister teaches me to ululate, rolls
her tongue in waves. Dips thin fingers inside
my mouth to pull out mine, stretches it long
and pinches the tip. Watch, we move tongues
like this. I hear the walls of our father's house
collapse and we become freeeeeelelelelelelelee.

On the ferry to Tangier I shriek across the sea.
Practice how to sound like a real woman. Old
aunties grab my buttocks, smush their breasts
against my back and sing lelelelelelelelelelelelelelelelelelelelelelelelelelelelelelelee.
Don't cover your mouth habibti! Only women
on the upper deck, only sea. We move tongues
like this to tell the waves stay back, tell men

stay back, tell the dead stay gone, tell runaway
wives stay gone. They turn me into wisteria
woman, limbs wrapped around poles and thighs
as they guide me. Throw back your head, epi
-glottis to the breeze. Salt air burns my throat's
hot membranes, catches on the tight knots of
my vocal chords. All my life I was told

women must swallow sand
unless we are sounding
a warning.

Hymen Hymn

hummmm
hum it
hum means "we"
in Urdu

we hummmm
hum hummm
"humesha" means always
always in Urdu

we always
hum humesha
hum it on a hymen
a hymn thin as a membrane

hum humesha humanghee
"humanghee" means harmony
we always harmonize
your mouth mucous membranes

on a half-moon membrane
reverberate in harmony
humesha humanghee hum
hummmm hum it

hum a hymen hymn
in two tongues one
language we hummmm
hummm hum it humesha

Ebola Cento

Oh mother, mother, where is happiness?
Fling your red dress faster and faster, dancer,
And say: *Sir were I you, as I should be,*
A very pestilence upon you fall!

Mango Pickle

Our sweet fruit is growing black
on the trees & Zafar keeps picking

his scabs. This heat tastes of gangrene,
honey sweet on the lips, vinegar

at the backs of our tongues.
Zafar said the boys pushed him,

knees, palms shredded across
the playground. My child

bandaged his skin, gritty & minced,
beneath polyester trousers—

I sniffed wounds sweating
a ripe pus. The mango farmer

has left the village—his wife said
he won't be coming back. She wrote

pestilence on the divorce paper,
the judge searched for a stamp

that said *blight*. Mangoes won't leave
the trees—their soggy stems keep swelling.

My Zafar whimpers in his sleep. I turn
black fruit to pickle, split hair

from stone, drain bitter juice
into jam jars.

Syndemics

First, I was born brown and then a woman.
Or the other way around: out came woman
& Muslim followed. My uncle called me
lighty as a term of endearment so maybe
I was not brown to begin with. Yes
I became brown in college. Become brown
every time I am in a room of White women,
pale into insignificance. Am woman only
with my feet in metal stirrups. Queer only
with my tongue inside another woman. First,
my shopping bag splits then a jar of olives
smashes open. First, I look for help in other
faces, then I spear olives with my nails.
When I open my mouth long vowels betray
my mother's village. First, I ask for a new
bag. First, I plead forgiveness. A brown
figure makes a scene, a crouching woman
grabs at olives, a hijaabi picks up cracked
glass. Which one of them is me?

If God Is a Virus

They are at the Million Man March
spreading legs and things, taking up
space at the corner of 12th Street
& Pennsylvania Avenue.

God is chanting about wombs, babies
& evolution, but it is not what you think.
Don't make assumptions about God.
God is not pro-life.

God is the security guard at the Planned
Parenthood on 4th Street NE, the one with
the plexiglass crucible where you yell
your name at God through a holey sheet
& God lets you in so a thing can be ripped
bloody and half grown off your cervix.

When the nurse sages your turmeric thighs
you cry Oh Bhagwan Oh Mara Allah, and
he lets you keep the speculum for puja. On
the way out, God is extra chatty—voice still
hoarse from all that chanting. God hands
you Kleenex and an evaluation form.

God wants the procedure to occur
before a man walks in with grenades
strapped to his beer belly threatens to
blow up all you heathens Muslims pagans

That doesn't happen—because there is
plexiglass & God. God is the security
guard working overtime because his
wife is pregnant & his youngest is anemic.

Because of that you walk out of the Planned
Parenthood without a neoplastic lesion,
go home and sleep off the local anesthetic.

My God Is a Virus

God is HPV and the anti-vaxxers
are the anti-Christ. God is cackling
because you won't give your kid
Gardasil in case it encourages sexual
activity. You would rather your kid
have cancer. That she meet God as a
seventeen-year-old in Planned Parenthood
in Washington DC. Her knickers
dotted with vinegar, cheap lube
& blood.

Ebola Cento

A bird flu over the city by night
And death shall be no more

Docile in his sexless dress
Death thou shalt die

NHS Zindabaad!

The coal miner's son delivered me through a gash
from comfy belly into Thatcher's ungloved hand.
Said This Is Your Religion Now—Let It Live.
So I raised a new fist and cried, NHS Zindabaad!

In this country where no body is well,
the lifeblood eats his midnight tea
in the hospital canteen: black pudding,
baked beans, and buttery toast before four

more wet babies are pulled, batteries
replaced, and finally the doctor loosens
his *pugg*, falls into a bleepless sleep. Whisper
in your dreams, NHS Zindabaad!

Once healers in our English land toiled
gardens in the Punjab, sailed ships across
the Atlantic so we could be born
in George Eliot's name. These sick streets

slick with immigrant electrolytes, pay slips
light, ash cash heavy. We burn joints, massage
soles, curse the politrickin' liars while we heel.
Abscesses need draining, bedpans need changing

—and the prime minister will never say, NHS
Zindabaad. In these dark cold days he keeps
trying to starve it, keeps trying to starve us
under budget cuts, my cala's blood sweetens

arteries tense with austerity and rage. I soothe her
with this story: in Amreeka the insulin would cost
your left leg and kalima finger. Swallow the bitter
pill, aunty, and plead with Allah: NHS Zindabaad!

Child of a nurse, lover of men, heed this poet's
warning, when it dies we die.
Let it live.
Let it live.
Let us live.

Acknowledgments

Reporting from West Africa was made possible by an award from the Pulitzer Center on Crisis Reporting. Thank you, Hannah Berk, for your work developing a teaching guide and workshops to accompany this book. My deepest appreciation to the Pulitzer Center team including Jon Sawyer, Tom Hundley, and Ann Peters for your continued support of my reporting and poetry.

Endless, deep, and lavender-scented gratitude to Nate Marshall, hands down one of the best poetry editors, for welcoming this book into the Break-Beat Poets series. Thanks to Maya Marshall, Nisha Bolsey, Kevin Coval, Jim Plank, and everyone at Haymarket for your work on this book. Thank you, Rayn Fox, for all of the support and energy you have poured into this manuscript and the editing process.

To my poetry community, Kundiman, and especially Third Dessert: thank you for your love, honesty, and guidance. All of my gratitude to agent extraordinaire, Lilly Ghahremani, who pours love and enthusiasm into every single project.

Thanks to the editors of the following magazines where earlier versions of poems were published:

"Self-Portrait as Virus"; "All the News That's Fit to Print"; "Liberia, Day Zero"; "Filovirus Phylogenetic Tree"; and "Misdiagnosis" appear in *Georgia Review*.

"Big Sister Teaches Me How to Ululate" appears in *Foundry*

"Lead Pipe–Dreams: Ghazal for Flint" appears in *Bateau Literary Magazine*

"The Queen's English" appears in *Ruminate Magazine*

"When the White Patient Asks for a White Doctor" appears in *Breakwater Review*

"Lady Doctor" appears in *Shallow Ends*

"Neologisms" appears in *Diode*

"Forty-One Surah Yaseens" appears in *Literary Review*

"Dua'a for Crossing Borders" appears in *Ellis Review*

"Hymen Hymn" appears in *Coal Hill Review*

"If God Is a Virus" appears in *Infection House*

"Syndemic" appears in *BOAAT Journal*

Notes

Surrogate Marker
borrows the phrase "carbolic halls" from the poem "Grace" by Roger Robinson.

Ebola News Cento
borrows lines from news reports about the 2014-2016 Ebola epidemic.

WHO Said
The first line is from a 1983 internal memo of the World Health Organization. The second line is from a November 20, 1986, United Nations address by World Health Organization Director-General Halfdan Mahler.

WHO Said
From internal memos of the World Health Organization.

What They Hear When They Listen to Your Heart
Racial bias in pain assessment and treatment recommendations, and false beliefs about biological differences between Blacks and Whites. Kelly M. Hoffman, Sophie Trawalter, Jordan R. Axt, and M. Norman Oliver. *Proceedings of the National Academy of Sciences of the United States of America*, April 19, 2016, 113 (16) 4296-4301; first published April 4, 2016 https://doi.org/10.1073/pnas.1516047113.

WHO Said
Comment by a World Health Organization official in the early days of the HIV/AIDS pandemic.

If God Is a Computer Virus
ILOVEYOU, also known as Love Letter or Love Bug, is a computer virus, created by Onel de Guzman, which infected more than ten million computers in 2000. ILOVEYOU replicated itself to infect other computers and spread much faster than previous computer viruses.

Ebola Cento
Lines for this cento are taken from "The Sonnet-Ballad" by Gwendolyn Brooks, "Mask" by Carl Sandburg, and "The Nun's Priest's Tale" from *The Canterbury Tales* by Geoffrey Chaucer.

Ebola Cento
Lines for this cento are taken from "Holy Numbers" by Fady Joudah, "Death, be not proud" (Holy Sonnet 10) by John Donne, and "First Communion" by Djuna Barnes.

NHS Zindabaad!
Zindabaad means "long live" and is a suffix in Urdu, Hindi, Bengali, Odia, and other Indian languages, derived from Farsi.

This poem references the chief architect of the United Kingdom's National Health Service, Aneurin "Nye" Bevan, the Welsh Labour Party politician who served as post-war minister of health. Son of a coal miner, Nye himself left school and mined coal at age 13. His father died from pneumoconiosis, a lung disease caused by inhalation of dust and smoke. Under Nye's watch, a national system of free medical care, funded by taxes, and available to all, was founded on July 5, 1948.

The following lines are adapted from, or inspired by, W.H. Auden:
"In this country where no body is well
Once healers in our English land
In these dark cold days
Child of a nurse, lover of men..."

Teaching Guide

Educators: Looking for a way to bring this book into your classroom? Visit pulitzercenter.org/ifgodisavirus for a free teaching guide developed by the Pulitzer Center for Crisis Reporting.

Resources include a lesson plan to introduce the book, discussion questions, writing prompts, and extension activities for language arts, journalism, social studies, and science classes.

This teaching guide supports students and educators in analyzing the poems in this book, and using *If God Is a Virus* to explore the ethics of documenting the world through poetry, journalism, science, and everyday observation.

Also by Seema Yasmin

Viral BS: Medical Myths and Why We Fall for Them (Johns Hopkins University Press, 2021)

Muslim Women Are Everything: Stereotype-Shattering Stories of Courage, Inspiration and Adventure (Harper Collins, 2020)

The Impatient Dr. Lange: One Man's Fight to End the Global HIV Epidemic (Johns Hopkins University Press, 2018)

About Haymarket Books

Haymarket Books is a radical, independent, nonprofit book publisher based in Chicago. Our mission is to publish books that contribute to struggles for social and economic justice. We strive to make our books a vibrant and organic part of social movements and the education and development of a critical, engaged, international left.

We take inspiration and courage from our namesakes, the Haymarket martyrs, who gave their lives fighting for a better world. Their 1886 struggle for the eight-hour day—which gave us May Day, the international workers' holiday—reminds workers around the world that ordinary people can organize and struggle for their own liberation. These struggles continue today across the globe—struggles against oppression, exploitation, poverty, and war.

Since our founding in 2001, Haymarket Books has published more than five hundred titles. Radically independent, we seek to drive a wedge into the risk-averse world of corporate book publishing. Our authors include Noam Chomsky, Arundhati Roy, Rebecca Solnit, Angela Y. Davis, Howard Zinn, Amy Goodman, Wallace Shawn, Mike Davis, Winona LaDuke, Ilan Pappé, Richard Wolff, Dave Zirin, Keeanga-Yamahtta Taylor, Nick Turse, Dahr Jamail, David Barsamian, Elizabeth Laird, Amira Hass, Mark Steel, Avi Lewis, Naomi Klein, and Neil Davidson. We are also the trade publishers of the acclaimed Historical Materialism Book Series and of Dispatch Books.

Also Available from Haymarket Books

Before the Next Bomb Drops: Rising Up from Brooklyn to Palestine
Remi Kanazi

Border and Rule: Global Migration, Capitalism, and the Rise of Racist Nationalism
Harsha Walia, afterword by Nick Estes, foreword by Robin D. G. Kelley

Crossfire: A Litany for Survival
Staceyann Chin, foreword by Jacqueline Woodson

Digging Our Own Graves
Coal Miners and the Struggle over Black Lung Disease
Barbara Ellen Smith, photography by Earl Dotter

Extracting Profit: Imperialism, Neoliberalism and the New Scramble for Africa
Lee Wengraf

My Mother Was a Freedom Fighter
Aja Monet

Reading Revolution: Shakespeare on Robben Island
Ashwin Desai

#SayHerName: Black Women's Stories of State Violence and Public Silence
African American Policy Forum, edited by Kimberlé Crenshaw
Foreword by Janelle Monáe

Text Messages: or How I Found Myself Time Traveling
Yassin "Narcy" Alsalman

We Still Here: Pandemic, Policing, Protest, and Possibility
Marc Lamont Hill, edited by Frank Barat
Foreword by Keeanga-Yamahtta Taylor